The Beginners Guide to Making Your Own Essential Oils

BY LINDSEY P

Complete Guide to Making Your Own Essential Oils from Scratch & To Improve Your Health and Well-Being

2nd Edition

The Beginners Guide to Making Your Own Essential Oils
2nd Edition

Copyright 2014 by Lindsey P - All rights reserved.

ISBN 978-1-329-21423-1

In no way is it legal to reproduce, duplicate, or transmit any part of this document in either electronic means or in printed format. Recording of this publication is strictly prohibited and any storage of this document is not allowed unless with written permission from the publisher. All rights reserved.

The Beginners Guide to Making Your Own Essential Oils
2nd Edition

Table Of Contents

Introduction 4

Chapter 1 What Are Essential Oils 6

Chapter 2 An Easy Way To Make Your Own Essential Oil At Home 8

Chapter 3 How To Make Your Own Essential Oil At Home Through Distillation 11

Chapter 4 How To Use Oil To Extract Essential Oil 13

Chapter 5 Essential Oils: Uses And Benefits 17

Chapter 6 List Of Essential Oils And Their Uses 24

Chapter 7 Aromatherapy for the Mind, Body and Spirit 28

Chapter 8 Aromatherapy Blends to Try 33

Chapter 9 Essential Oil for Medical Purposes 44

Chapter 10 Create Your Own Products Using Essential Oils 55

Conclusion 73

Check Out My Other Books 74

The Beginners Guide to Making Your Own Essential Oils 2nd Edition

Introduction

I want to thank you and congratulate you for purchasing the book, The Beginners Guide To Making Your Own Essential Oils: Complete Guide To Making Your Own Essential Oils From Scratch & To Improve Your Health And Well-Being.

This book contains proven steps and strategies on how to make your very own essentials oils to keep you healthy and away from many diseases and sicknesses.

Since the beginning of time, aromatherapy has been used by our ancestors to promote health, for medical practice and for personal hygiene. Aromatherapy uses essential oils extracted from flowers, stems, leaves, barks and other parts of a plant. These essential oils are believed to enhance physical as well as psychological well-being.

The aroma of these essential oils is believed to stimulate brain function when inhaled. Essential oils are also absorbed through the skin easily, wherein they promote well-being and healing by travelling through the bloodstream.

More and more people are discovering the medicinal benefits of aromatherapy, which is why it is gaining popularity really fast. Aromatherapy is used in various applications including increased cognitive function, enhanced mood and pain relief.

The Beginners Guide to Making Your Own Essential Oils
2nd Edition

There are numerous essential oils and aromatherapy products available. Each of them has their own healing properties.

This book explains what essential oils are and how they are made. Inside, you will also discover various essential oils and the benefits that they offer. You can use this book as a guide on how to use aromatherapy and which essential oil is best to use for a specific condition.

Thanks again for purchasing this book, I hope you enjoy it!

The Beginners Guide to Making Your Own Essential Oils 2nd Edition

Chapter 1

What Are Essential Oils

Essential oils are extracted from leaves, flowers, barks, stems, roots and other parts of a plant, commonly by steam. Essential oils are commonly clear but may also have amber, yellow or deep blue color. Essential oils are also referred to as essences since they contain the true essence of the plant where they are extracted from. Although essential oils have pleasing aromatic scents, they are different from fragrance oils.

Unlike fragrance oils, essential oils are pure and do not contain artificial fragrances or substances, that is why fragrance oils are not suitable for aromatherapy. Essential oils are used for its therapeutic benefits since the beginning of recorded history. These essential oils are usually inhaled or applied to the skin for absorption. History has proven the psychological and physical therapeutic benefits of essentials oils, although no scientific evidence has proven it.

Since essential oils are either inhaled or applied directly to the skin, you should take time to check if you have any allergic reactions to any of them. Apply a small amount to the side of your hand and wait for a few hours for any allergic reactions. Moreover, if you are allergic to the source plant, fruit or seed, chances are, you are also allergic to the essential oil extracted from it.

The Beginners Guide to Making Your Own Essential Oils
2nd Edition

Although they are called "essential oils", they are not really oils. Unlike actual oil, essential oils do not contain fatty acids which make them actual oil. Furthermore, essential oils are volatile and they evaporate when left uncovered. Essential oils are often diluted in carrier oils such as grape seed oil, sweet almond oil and apricot kernel oil. You can buy essential oils individually bottled in small bottles. Most essential oils are sold as blends of various essential oils such as the Thieves essential oil. This essential oil is a combination of clove, lemon, cinnamon, eucalyptus and rosemary essential oils.

Chapter 2

An Easy Way to Make Your Own Essential Oil At Home

Essential oils are generally extracted from plants through distillation, commonly using steam. But other processes are also used such as solvent extraction, florasols extraction and expression. Essential oils are greatly used in perfumes, soaps and cosmetics. They are also used to flavor food and drinks and to add scent to household cleaning products and incense.

One of the most popular and easiest essential oil to make at home is the orange essential oil. Orange peels usually end up in the garbage and are just wasted. Instead of buying expensive scents, you can make your very own citrus scent at home without spending too much. Furthermore, making your own essential oil means you are guaranteed to be using a 100% natural product, free from harmful chemicals.

This procedure is an example of extracting essential oil using alcohol.

All you need are the following:

    Orange peels (remove most of the white pith as possible)

    Glass jar or glass bottle with a tight lid

The Beginners Guide to Making Your Own Essential Oils
2nd Edition

  Vodka (No need for the expensive ones. Any cheap vodka will do)

  Undenatured Ethyl alcohol (as a substitute for the Vodka)

  Coffee filter (cheesecloth or muslin will do)

  Paper towel (muslin or cheesecloth can also be used as a substitute)

Dry your orange peels in a warm, dry place but away from direct sunlight until they are hard and dry. It usually takes 2 days for this but you can cut the orange peels into smaller pieces to help dry them faster.

Place the dried orange peels into the glass jar or bottle. Place the bottle of vodka or undenatured ethyl alcohol into a bowl of hot tap water for a few minutes then pour it into the jar/bottle of dried orange peels until they are all soaked. Cover the jar/bottle tightly and shake it vigorously for 2 to 3 minutes. Do this three to four times a day for 3 days or more. The more you shake the mixture and the longer you leave the orange peels soaked, the more oil you can extract.

Using a coffee filter or cheesecloth, strain the orange peels into a bowl. Cover it with cheesecloth or paper towel. Do not let the towel/cloth fall into the liquid as it will seep it and you will lose your essential oil.

Let the liquid sit for a few days in a cool, dark and clean area until all the alcohol has evaporated. Now you have

The Beginners Guide to Making Your Own Essential Oils
2nd Edition

pure orange essential oil that you can use for fragrance, soaps, candles, lotion, potpourris or aromatic waters.

When extracting essential oil from leaves or flowers using undenatured ethyl alcohol or vodka, the process is almost the same as above. The only difference is, when you strain the flowers/leaves from the mixture, you need to gently press them to release more oil. Furthermore, while you are soaking them in alcohol or vodka, you can add more leaves or flowers until you are able to reach your desired strength for your essential oil.

The Beginners Guide to Making Your Own Essential Oils 2nd Edition

Chapter 3

How to Make Your Own Essential Oil At Home through Distillation

The most popular way of extracting essential oil from plants is through distillation. Normally, you need an apparatus called the still to be able to collect essential oil from plants. But, if you do not have distillation equipment and you want to create your own essential, it is still possible. The yield may not be as great as when you are using a still and the process may be longer but it's a great alternative.

You will need a crock pot, some distilled water, air-tight glass container, bowl and cheesecloth. This procedure is very simple but it takes time.

- Decide what plant material you want to extract essential oil from. Dry your plant material. Make sure not to over dry them and do not place them under direct sunlight as it may lose some of its essential oils.

- Place your dried plant material into the crock pot and fill it with distilled water until all the plant material is soaked.

- Cook in low heat for 24 hours. Do not attempt to increase the heat to make the process faster as it will affect the quality and yield of the essential oil.

The Beginners Guide to Making Your Own Essential Oils
2nd Edition

- Leave crock pot open until cool. Cover with cloth and let it sit in a cool, dry place for a week. You will see oil separating on top of the water in the crock pot. Collect the oil off and place it in a dark, tightly covered container.

- Cover the container with cheesecloth and allow the rest of the water to evaporate. This will take about a week.

- You now have your very own essential oil made possible through distillation at home.

Another distillation method that can be done at home is by grounding up your dried plant material. Use a cotton or linen bag as a container for your ground plant material for cooking. Make sure to tie the bag shut so that no plant material falls off during the process.

Put some distilled water in a crock pot, enough to soak up the bag of plant material. Bring it to a boil. When the water is already boiling, reduce the heat to low and let it simmer for 24 hours.

Let the water cool. You will notice some oil on the surface of the water. Collect the oil and place in a clean, dry, dark glass container. Squeeze the bag unto the water in the crock pot and collect the oil from the surface.

Cover the glass container with clean cloth (cheesecloth or cotton preferably). Let it sit in a cool, dry place for a week to allow the excess water to evaporate.

You can now enjoy your very own essential oil.

The Beginners Guide to Making Your Own Essential Oils 2nd Edition

Chapter 4
How to Use Oil to Extract Essential Oil

Extracting essential oil using is very and can be done from home. It is most ideal to use almond oil, Jojoba oil or rapeseed for this process. Do not use a metal container when using oils to extract essential oils from plant materials as it will affect the quality of the essential oil. Use non-metallic containers only such as ceramic crock or glass containers.

This process is best used for herbs and flowers such as rosemary, lavender, rose or the likes. You may or may not dry your herb or flowers. It all depends on you. Drying can reduce the amount of essential oil from your herb/flower but it can help increase your yield per batch as you will be able to cramp in more herbs/flowers per batch.

Things you will need:

Large glass bottle

Extracting oil (rapeseed, almond or jojoba)

Cheesecloth

Procedure:

Fill half of the large glass bottle with your extracting oil (carrier oil) such as jojoba, rapeseed or almond). Put as much herbs/flowers/leaves into the glass bottle. Make

The Beginners Guide to Making Your Own Essential Oils
2nd Edition

sure that all the plant materials are completely submerged into the oil. Cover the glass tightly with its lid and let sit for 24 hours in a cool, dark, clean area.

Shake the mixture from time to time within three days. You can do this three to four times each day. Shaking will help extract more oil from the plant material.

After three days, strain the plant material. Use a ceramic bowl to catch the oil from the glass bottle. You can add more plant materials into the oil if the scent is not strong enough for you. Remember, you have to let it sit for 24 hours and repeat all the process after that.

Place your extracted essential oil in a dark, clean container. This essential oil is ready to use.

Another way of extracting essential oil from a plant material using oil is by slow cooking. Here's how to do it:

- In a crock pot, place 2 cups of olive oil (jojoba, rapeseed or almond) and mix ½ ounce of plant material (flowers, leaves, herbs, etc) into it.

- Slow cook the mixture in low heat for up to 6 hours. You may stir the mixture a few times to ensure that the plant materials are completely soaked into the carrier oil (olive oil, jojoba, rapeseed, almond).

- Leave the crock pot open to cool the mixture.

- Strain the oil mixture using an unbleached cheese cloth. Use a ceramic bowl to place the oil while straining.

The Beginners Guide to Making Your Own Essential Oils
2nd Edition

- Place the essential oil in a dark, clean, tightly covered glass bottle and use sparingly.

Another easy way of extracting essential oil from plant materials using is by grounding the plant materials and soaking them in carrier oils. This process takes a long time of waiting but it's fairly easy to do.

First, dry your plant material. Do not expose your plant material in direct sunlight as it will lose most of its essential oils. Dry in a dark, cool place for about 2 days. Do not over dry. When the plant material is already wilted and dried, it's ready to be grounded.

After grinding the plant material, take one tablespoon and place it in a clear, glass bottle or jar. Add ½ cup of carrier oil (olive oil, rapeseed, almond, jojoba) and ½ teaspoon white vinegar. Stir to combine all the ingredients. Cover the glass bottle/jar and leave it in a warm, sunny area for three weeks. Make sure to place the bottle in an area where there is plenty sunlight. Shake the bottle two to three times a day for three weeks.

Strain the mixture and place your essential oil in a dark, glass container. Please note that essential oils are very pure so they must be used in small amounts only.

To ensure that you are not allergic to any essential oils, perform the skin patch test. Place a small amount of essential oil on the side of your palm. Wait for a few hours. If no irritation, itchiness or swelling occurs, you are not allergic to the essential oil and you may continue using it. In general, if you are allergic to the herb, flower

The Beginners Guide to Making Your Own Essential Oils
2nd Edition

or fruit of a certain plant, you are most likely allergic to its essential oil as well.

Chapter 5
Essential Oils: Uses and Benefits

The use of essential oils and making your own at home can be very fun, fulfilling and beneficial therapeutically. Always remember that essential oils are not meant to be swallowed or ingested. There may be some essential oils that are safe to ingest, but even so, you still need to consult an expert before ingesting any essential oils.

Essential oils are commonly inhaled. For first timers, you can place one to two drops of your desired essential oil in a piece of tissue and carefully inhale the scent. Those who are already veterans in using essential oils usually place a small amount of essential oil on their palm and rub it a little, and then they cover their nose with their palm and inhale the aroma of the essential oil.

When you are suffering from colds or influenza, the best way to treat your condition with essential oils is through steam inhalation. Pour 2 cups of boiled water in a bowl and add 3 to 7 drops of essential oil into it. You may lessen the number of drops if you are using essential oils with strong scents that may irritate your mucus membranes. Some of these essential oils include thyme, rosemary, cinnamon, pine eucalyptus, cajuput and others. Do not place your nose too near the bowl. Put at least about 10 to 12 inches gap between the bowl and your nose. Inhale the steam gradually and carefully. Do not inhale constantly as it may irritate your nose. If you feel

The Beginners Guide to Making Your Own Essential Oils 2nd Edition

any discomfort or irritation, discontinue use right away. This can be done anytime, day or night.

Please note that too much inhalation of essential oils can cause dizziness, vertigo, lethargy, nausea and headaches. Although essential oils are greatly used to treat respiratory problems and sinuses, you must take precaution when using them. Do not use over 10 drops. Aside from hot water, you may also use diffusers or hot compress for inhalation.

Essential oils are also great for making your room smell fresh. To expel any unwanted smell in your house, you may sprinkle a few drops of essential oils in your trash can, drain, vacuum bag filter or laundry wash. You may also add a few drops on your tissue before you keep them in your cabinet. Please take note that essential oils are flammable. Do not place them near fire or too much heat.

Essential oils are also great insect repellents. Essential oils of citronella, peppermint and lavender are natural insect repellents. To prevent insects from infesting your household, place a few drops on a cotton ball and place it on your doorway, windows and other areas where you frequently see insects. If you are a pet owner, some essential oils are not suitable for pets. Some of these essential oils include anise, garlic, juniper, horseradish, clove leaf or clove bud, thyme, Wintergreen, yarrow and others.

On the contrary, there are also some essential oils that are used for pets, especially for dogs due to their calming effects. Most common of these are chamomile, eucalyptus,

The Beginners Guide to Making Your Own Essential Oils
2nd Edition

lavender, ginger, myrrh, rose, valerian, cedarwood atlas, ravensare and others. Essential oils are usually used for pet baths and for calming the pet's nerves through diffusion.

Remember that your pet cannot tell you if it is or is not working. Always check for signs of irritation as excessive scratching, too much whining, sniffing and nervousness. If any of these signs are present, discontinue use.

Either for humans or for pets always dilute your essential oil. For pets, essential oils are best diluted at 25% of human formula. Never use essential oils internally for your pets. Size matters for essential oils. Smaller pets should be given smaller amount of essential oil. But even if your pet is huge, let's say a horse; less is still better with essential oils. Birds and fish should never be given essential oils. Birds are highly sensitive and cannot tolerate essential oils just as fish cannot tolerate floral waters or oils.

Essential oils are also greatly used for a relaxing massage. Do not use any essential oil that is not diluted as it may cause skin irritations. Use 1 ounce of carrier oil such as almond oil and add 10 to 20 drops of essential oil. Do not apply on the genitals and near the eyes.

Essential oils are also popularly used for soaps, shampoos, lotions, shower gels, facial toners and perfumes for their great aroma and therapeutic benefits.

If you are experiencing circulatory problems, skin problems, respiratory symptoms, menstrual pain, muscle pain or stress and nervous tension, an aromatic bath will

The Beginners Guide to Making Your Own Essential Oils
2nd Edition

give you great relief. Please be aware that essential oils should be mixed with either salt or emulsifier like sesame oil or milk before they can be safely dispersed into the water. Essential oils will float on water if not mixed with salt or emulsifier and will directly get into the skin which can cause irritations.

Aromatic bath uses warm water and essential oils that are not mixed with salt or emulsifier can cause dermotoxicity especially if the essential oil used is of a heating nature. For safety purposes, avoid spicy oils in your bath. These essential oils include thyme, tulsi, oregano and cinnamon oil. Also, avoid phototoxic oils such as bergamot oil and citrus oils. Essential oils with specific irritant potential such as lemongrass should also be avoided. Essential oils that are generally considered mild for use in baths are:

- Lavender oil
- Clary Sage oil
- Rose oil
- Geranium oil
- Frankincense oil
- Sandalwood oil
- Eucalyptus oil
- Cedar oil
- Fir oil

The Beginners Guide to Making Your Own Essential Oils
2nd Edition

- Pine oil

- Pinon pine essential oil

- Spruce oil

- Juniper oil

Combine 5 to 10 drops of essential oil in ½ to 1 cup of salt or emulsifier and add it into your warm bath. Do not soak too long in aromatic water. The ideal soaking time is between 10 to 15 minutes only. Soaking too long under aromatic baths may cause skin irritation and other symptoms such as headache and nausea.

If you suffer from dysmenorrhea or menstrual cramps, skin problems and muscle aches or if you have a wound or a bruise, you can use essential oil (lavender, thieves, Melrose) compress for relief. Just add 10 drops of essential oil in 4oz of warm water and soak a clean cloth in it. Wring the cloth gently and place it on the affected area. Repeat the process for 10 to 15 minutes.

For relief from inflammation, you may use the following essential oils for your compress:

- Wintergreen – This essential oil has a warming effect. Its methyl salicylate and cortisone-like effect reduces inflammation and pain in the muscles and joints.

- Helichrysum – This essential oil has powerful anti-inflammatory properties making it ideal for cuts and bruises. It also helps boost circulation and cleanses the blood.

- Clove – This essential oil helps relieve pain due to arthritis and rheumatism. It has anti-infectious properties as well as anti-inflammatory, anesthetic and antiseptic properties which also make it ideal for wounds, scrapes and bruises.

- Peppermint – For pain, peppermint essential oil is great. It has pain blocking properties, antispasmodic and anti-inflammatory properties. It provides cooling and soothing effects and it also dilates the respiratory system.

- Palo Santo – Due to its anticoagulant and anti-inflammatory properties, this essential oil is excellent for relieving tired muscles and joints. It is also rich in limonene, an antioxidant.

- Lemon – Essential oil extracted from lemon has antiseptic properties which make it great for wounds and cuts. It also has immune-stimulating properties which uplifts your mood.

- Copal/Copaiba – This essential oil has excellent anti-inflammatory properties which are good for wounds, cuts and bruises. It is also an antiseptic, antibacterial and analgesic. Furthermore, Copaiba/Copal essential oil helps boost the respiratory, nervous and cardiovascular systems.

The Beginners Guide to Making Your Own Essential Oils
2nd Edition

Essential oils are also used for massage due to their calming and warming effects as well as their therapeutic benefits. Take note that essential oils are pure and must be diluted in carrier oils before use. For adults, it is ideal to place 12 drops of essential oil in an ounce of carrier oil. For children under 12 years old, it is generally safe to use 6 drops of essential oil in an ounce of carrier oil. You may lessen the number of drops for the essential oils especially if you are just starting.

The Beginners Guide to Making Your Own Essential Oils 2nd Edition

Chapter 6

List of Essential Oils and Their Uses

There are so many essential oils out in the market and there are even more that are yet to be discovered. Below is a quick guide to essential oils and their uses.

- Basil – This essential oil is antiviral, antibacterial, antispasmodic and anti-inflammatory. It is also a muscle relaxant, stimulant, decongestant and antiseptic. Due to its therapeutic properties, basil essential oil is often used to treat migraines, muscle aches and pains, mental fatigue, anxiety, depression, throat and lung infections, bronchitis, menstrual cramps, dandruff and insect bites. It can also be used as an insect repellant for flies and mosquitoes.

    You may dilute it in carrier oil such as vegetable or coconut oil. A 50:50 dilution is ideal, meaning one part basil essential oil is to one part carrier oil. You may apply the diluted basil essential oil in the problem areas or inhale it by placing 1 to 2 drops on the palm of your hand rubbing it lightly. If you are asthmatic, do not inhale any essential oil. Instead, place it on the sole of your feet. You may also diffuse it by using the candle method or the steam method.

The Beginners Guide to Making Your Own Essential Oils
2nd Edition

- Bergamot – Bergamot is known for its relaxing and uplifting effect and has a sweet and fruity scent. It is used to help fight addiction and to relieve stress, anxiety and depression. It is also know to relieve infections such as herpes and vaginal candida as well as cold sores, urinary tract infections and respiratory infections. You may use diluted Bergamot essential oil for massage or apply topically on the affected area. You can also diffuse it or inhale it by adding a few drops on your palm.

- Clary Sage – The sharp, grassy and spicy aroma of Clary Sage essential oil helps relax the mind. It helps prevent hair loss by boosting hair growth. It is an antioxidant, astringent and antiseptic making it effective in preventing wrinkles and keeps skin healthy (for dry and oily skin). It helps relieve menstrual problems and PMS, pre-menopausal symptoms, insomnia, impotence, hemorrhoids, bronchitis, high cholesterol and kidney disorders.

- Chamomile – Chamomile essential oil can tone the skin through continued use. It is also a known anti-depressant and reduces nervousness.

- Cinnamon – For the relief of joint pains and improved circulation, cinnamon essential oil is greatly advised. It also helps reduce nervousness by calming the nerves.

- Cucumber – Essential oil extracted from cucumber is an excellent detoxifier and skin moisturizer. It also helps reduce puffiness of the eyes. The calming effect of cucumber essential oil is great for relaxing the mind and body.

- Eucalyptus – This essential oil is effective in killing lice. Dilute one part eucalyptus essential oil to one part coconut oil and apply to hair. Leave for 5 to 10 minutes only. Rinse off with water or shampoo. It also eases joint and muscle pains and clears respiratory passages.

- Jasmine – This is a must-have for girls. Jasmine essential oil reduces scars and helps relieve PMS symptoms. It is also effective in relieving muscle spasms and for treating dry and sensitive skin.

- Lavender – This essential oil is best known for its calming effect making it an effective treatment for insomnia and stress. It also reduces symptoms of PMS.

- Lemon – Lemon essential oil is known to clear respiratory passages making it effective for the treatment of colds and other respiratory problems. The antibacterial and antiseptic properties of lemon essential oil also make it an effective treatment for acne. It also boosts the immune system, treat dandruff and helps lower down fever.

- Orange – Essential oil from orange has anti-inflammatory properties which relieve pain and inflammation. It is also an anti-depressant and an aphrodisiac.

The Beginners Guide to Making Your Own Essential Oils
2nd Edition

- Peppermint – For fast relief of headache, peppermint essential oil is highly recommended. It also relieves nausea and decreases indigestion. It also eases clogged nose and relieves other respiratory problems.

- Sage – Sage essential oil heals wounds, fights infections and calms upset stomach.

Always remember to store your essential oils in a cool dry place and away from direct sunlight and heat as it may lose its potency and its quality can be compromised.

Chapter 7
Aromatherapy for the Mind, Body and Spirit

Aromatherapy is popular in spas and wellness centers because of their many benefits. Aromatherapy refers to the art and science of using extracted essential oil to harmonize, balance and promote overall wellness. The scientific aspect of aromatherapy comes from distinguishing the difference in aroma chemicals of each essential oil. Aromatherapy has many benefits to the mind, body and spirit.

Benefits to the mind

Essential oils can stimulate part of the brain that is responsible for emotions. It triggers olfactory nerves in the nostrils and sends the impression to the limbic system where there are stored memories and perceived emotions. The limbic system can then release chemicals like serotonin, which alleviates anxiety, as well as endorphins that can reduce pain.

Directly inhaling essential oil is very pleasurable and helps you achieve emotional balance quickly. You can also diffuse it in the air while being massaged or while taking a bath for a gradual treatment approach.

Stress relief

The Beginners Guide to Making Your Own Essential Oils
2nd Edition

Aromatherapy is one of the sought after relaxation treatments. Many studies show just how much aromatherapy can help people relax and unwind. Essential oils are more popularly used as a home remedy for stress and anxiety. It is simple and easy to use and the effects can be immediate.

Antidepressant capacity

Essential oils are also useful when it comes to eliminating feelings of depression. Prescribed antidepressants can have serious side effects so some people opt to try complementary treatments like aromatherapy instead.

Memory enhancement

One of the most frightening diseases that affect middle aged to elderly is memory loss and inability to retain short-term memory. Alzheimer's disease is still an incurable disease, but you can help slow down its progress by using several treatments like aromatherapy. Studies show that regularly attending aromatherapy sessions can improve memory capacity for a short time after the treatment. Sage essential oil is the most recommended essential oil for memory boosting effects.

Benefits to the body

Essential oils are absorbed into the skin quickly. It passes through different cells and into sebaceous glands where it mixes with the skin's natural oil. The chemical properties

The Beginners Guide to Making Your Own Essential Oils
2nd Edition

of the oil can have detoxifying, energizing, calming or balancing effects on the body.

Boost energy levels

Everyone can benefit from energy booster several times a day. However, stimulants like coffee and energy drinks have serious effects on the body. A healthy diet and exercise can boost you energy. Aromatherapy is also used to increase energy and improve mood. Many essential oils can stimulate circulation without the side effects of other stimulants. The best oils to use for energy boost include clove, sage, jasmine, pepper, tea tree, angelica, cinnamon and cardamom.

Better healing and recovery

Essential oils can help speed up the recovery of wounds. Essential oils can increase the blood flow to external and internal wounds. The antimicrobial properties of the essential oil can also help protect the body from infection. Some of the essential oils can do more than just healing wounds. They can also help relieve discomfort usually experienced during the healing process like redness and itchiness.

Headaches

Headaches can range from mild to severe. The really bad ones can prevent people from doing anything productive. Commercial medicine can be very expensive and it has several side effects. Aromatherapy can be a wonderful treatment for headache. It even has additional benefits like stress reduction that can prevent headaches in the future. Some essential oils used for migraine includes peppermint, sandalwood, rosemary and eucalyptus essential oil. You can make a blend out of these oils and spread the mixture in your scalp, temples and neck.

Get better sleep

Sleep deprivation has serious mental and physical effects. Not getting enough rest can leave you unproductive and sluggish throughout the day. Fortunately, essential oils are great to use to improve your sleeping pattern and can help you readapt to your circadian rhythms so that you get enough rest at the appropriate time. Essential oils that have sedative effects include sandalwood, ylang ylang, sweet marjoram, jasmine, chamomile and lavender.

Boosts immune system

Most medical professionals agree that prevention is better than cure when it comes to disease and illness. Aromatherapy can help boost your immune system if you know how to use it properly. Essential oils that have antibacterial, antifungal and antimicrobial effects can protect you from many illness and infection that can damage your system. This benefit of aromatherapy has been widely studied. The most effective oils to improve your immune system include oregano, lemon, cinnamon, peppermint, eucalyptus and frankincense.

Pain Relief

Analgesic is a popular medicine to relive pain. However, it can also cause nausea, decreased appetite, kidney damage, stomach ulcer and constipation if it is used for a long period of time. Pain relief is one of the useful benefits of aromatherapy. It can gradually reduce the pain while relaxing your senses at the same time.

Digestion

Aromatherapy can also treat some digestive issues. It can help ease constipation, bloating and indigestion. It can even speed up metabolism and help you lose weight even while at rest. Citrus essential oils have been known to treat digestive issues. You can combine it with other oils like ginger, clary sage, fennel and chamomile for better results.

Benefits to the spirit

Essential oils have been around for several centuries because ancient cultures believe that these oils have spiritual and mystical properties that can help them connect with the Divine. Ancient people perceived essential oils as the spirit of the plants that are contained in a jar. You can try using essential oils when meditating and praying.

Essential oil and aromatherapy have wonderful benefits to every level of your being. It can help enhance your mind, body and spirit. Aromatherapy is one of the most creative ways to harness the power of essential oils.

The Beginners Guide to Making Your Own Essential Oils
2nd Edition

Chapter 8

Aromatherapy Blends to Try

After learning how to make you own essential oil through different processes, you are ready to use them in aromatherapy. Most beginners are more comfortable in using just one essential oil at a time. As you become more comfortable with the process, you can start trying different essential oil blends too.

Blending essential oils for beginners

There are companies that sell pre-blended essential oil in a bottle. However, it is easy to make your own synergy blends and personalize them to suit your needs and preference. Synergy blends refer to combinations of essential oil that can work together to provide a particular benefit.

Before you start blending essential oils, you first have to determine the purpose of the oil blend. Also, determine how you will use the oils. For example, you want to create an energizing blend, you will have to determine if you want to apply it topically or add it to your bath water. You will have to use essential oils that are safe for the skin and dilute properly using carrier oils and other liquid.

Step 1: Choose oils that have the properties that you need

After determining the type of essential oil that you want to make, you need to gather all the essential oils that you are

The Beginners Guide to Making Your Own Essential Oils 2nd Edition

going to use. Go over the benefits of each essential oil and choose the main ingredients that you will use.

Step 2: Blending oils based on categories and notes

Most beginners find this part difficult. The trick is to choose the oils based on their category and note. This is to ensure that your aromatherapy blend smells nice.

Essential oils are categorized based on their aromas. Oils that are from the same category tend to blend well together.

Categories:

Woodsy- Cedar and Pine

Herbaceous- Basil, Marjoram and Rosemary

Medicinal- Tea tree, Eucalyptus and Cajuput

Oriental- Patchouli and Ginger

Floral- Jasmine, Lavender and Neroli

Earthy- Patchouli, Oakmos, Vetiver

Minty- Spearmint and Peppermint

Spicy- Cinnamon, Nutmeg and Clove

Citrus- Lime, Orange and Lemon

How to blend categories:

Woodsy oils tend to blend well with other categories

The Beginners Guide to Making Your Own Essential Oils
2nd Edition

Mint oils are best paired with earthy, woodsy, herbaceous and citrus oils

Floral blends can be combined with citrus, woodsy and spicy essential oils

Spicy and oriental blends are great to pair with citrus, floral and oriental oils

These guidelines can help beginners create their own aromatherapy blend.

Essential oil notes

How quickly the essential oil evaporates depends on its 'note'. You might notice that essential oil can smell differently after several hours. The notes are based on the musical scale and are categorized as top, middle and base notes.

Top notes include basil, spearmint, bergamot, lemon, peppermint, eucalyptus, lemongrass and grapefruit. The middle notes are cypress, tea tree, clary sage, pine and rosemary. The base notes are ginger, myrrh, vanilla, sandalwood, frankincense and helichrysum.

After initial application, you will usually smell the combination of all the oils. The top note will evaporate first and you will be left with the middle and base note. The middle note will also evaporate after the first 2-3 hours and you will only smell the base note.

It is advisable for beginners to start with only three oils and choose one oil from each note. You can start adding

The Beginners Guide to Making Your Own Essential Oils 2nd Edition

essential oil to your blend once you become more comfortable.

Step 3: Blending and testing oil blends

For beginners, you can start with only just 10 drops of oil. This lets you experiment without wasting so much of your precious essential oil. Remember that you are only blending essential oils in this step and are not diluting it in carrier oils just yet. As a general tip, you can use the 30,50,20 rule where you use 30% top note oil, 50% middle note oil and 20% base oil.

Step 4: Let it rest

The fourth step is generally the easiest part. Once you have combined your essential oils, you need to set it aside for 1-2 days. The rest period allows the chemical properties of the oil to mix together.

Step 5: Test your blend

After the resting period, you are ready to smell the mixture. You can try diluting it in carrier oil if you find the scent too strong. Once you like the scent, you can make more of it in larger quantities. If you are not satisfied with the blend, you can start all over again and try other essential oils.

Balancing Blends

Lavender Balancing Blend

The Beginners Guide to Making Your Own Essential Oils
2nd Edition

Lavender is one of the most popular and useful essential oils. Lavender is also very versatile and you can mix it with other oils to improve its scent quality.

7 drops lavender oil

1 drop patchouli oil

7 drops bergamot oil

1 drop juniper berry oil

Soothing Back Blend

This is a great aromatherapy blend that can sooth back and butt pain.

30 drops German chamomile oil

6 drops peppermint oil

2 drops clove oil

10 drops Roman chamomile oil

4 drops wintergreen oil

Red Cedarwood Blend

Cedarwood has a subtle woody scent that can promote balance. You can mix it with the strong floral scent of rose.

20 drops cedarwood oil

20 drops myrrh oil

30 drops rose oil

The Beginners Guide to Making Your Own Essential Oils
2nd Edition

20 drops sandalwood oil

10 drops patchouli oil

Wintertime Blend

This is a wonderful winter season blend that is dominated by pine and fir needle scents.

10 drops cedarwood oil

15 drops fir needle oil

20 drops sandalwood oil

25 drops bergamot orange oil

30 drops juniper berry oil

Patchouli Personal Blend

This blend has a distinct floral aroma that you can adjust to suit your preference. You can increase the amount of rose essential oil for a lighter fragrance or add clove and cinnamon for a spicier scent.

6 drops patchouli oil

10 drops bergamot oil

4 drops rose oil

Energizing Blends

Uplifting Lemon Blend

Citrus essential oils have wonderful energizing effects on the body. It can help improve your mood too.

The Beginners Guide to Making Your Own Essential Oils 2nd Edition

20 drops lemon oil

25 drops neroli oil

20 drops tangerine oil

35 drops lavender oil

Sweet Clarity Blend

This energizing blend is not too strong or overpowering. It can even blend well with sweet scent oils, making it pleasant and energizing.

20 drops peppermint oil

35 drops lavender oil

20 drops spearmint oil

25 drops lemon oil

Summertime Blend

This essential oil blend is inspired the by the scent of summer. It is great to use outdoors.

8 drops eucalyptus oil

4 drops grapefruit oil

4 drops grapefruit oil

8 drops eucalyptus oil

Stimulating Blend

The Beginners Guide to Making Your Own Essential Oils
2nd Edition

This simple but very effective energizing blend is perfect for you if you want to experience the soothing effects immediately.

3 drops eucalyptus oil

3 drops sweet orange oil

10 drops peppermint oil

2 drops ginger oil

Purifying & Energizing Blend

Use this blend to increase your energy and motivation during your workout.

8 drops lemon oil

5 drops rosemary oil

8 drops peppermint oil

Romantic Blends

Vanilla Love Blend

Vanilla has a sensual and romantic scent that blends well with sweet and floral oils.

20 drops vanilla oil

1 drop cardamom oil

2 drops sweet orange oil

3 drops rose otto oil

The Beginners Guide to Making Your Own Essential Oils
2nd Edition

Love Massage Blend

This is a great blend for massage. It can also provide relaxation benefits.

30 drops rose otto oil

5 drops sandalwood oil

10 drops vanilla oil

Seduction Blend

This blend is a combination of exotic and sweet scent that can tickle your senses.

1 drop jasmine oil

1 drop patchouli oil

2 drops vanilla oil

Love Potion Blend

Use this romantic blend to evoke the romantic mood that you desire.

55 drops rose absolute oil

6 drops ylang ylang

1 drop clove bud oil

Relaxing Blend

The Beginners Guide to Making Your Own Essential Oils 2nd Edition

Absolute Bliss

This aromatherapy blend has wonderful relaxing properties from the coriander, bergamot and lavender oils. This is perfect to use after a strenuous day.

22 drops lavender oil

6 drops bergamot

6 drops coriander oil

2 drops patchouli oil

Holiday Head Soother

This is a great blend to use if you are feeling stressed from all the things that you need to accomplish.

12 drops frankincense oil

2 drops lavender oil

3 drops peppermint oil

Warm and Cozy Blend

This soothing blend is very effective in relaxing your tired muscles.

10 drops bergamot oil

2 drops cinnamon leaf oil

6 drops lavender oil

½ tsp sweet almond oil

The Beginners Guide to Making Your Own Essential Oils
2nd Edition

Ylang Citrus Relaxing Blend

The combination of bergamot and mandarin adds a fresh scent to this strong floral blend.

15 drops ylang ylang oil

40 drops bergamot oil

45 drops mandarin orange oil

Luxurious Relaxing Blend

Create a luxurious blend that can soothe your tired muscles after a long day.

3 drops lavender oil

3 drops eucalyptus oil

2 tbsp sweet almond oil

3 drops peppermint oil

Chapter 9
Essential Oil for Medicinal Purpose

Essential oils are popularly used in aromatherapy because of their many benefits. Essential oils can help you stay alert during the day and help you relax and unwind at night. Hospitals are also experimenting on the effects of essential oils to help patients relax. Another great benefit of essential oils is the treatment for common health problems.

Asthma Treatment

Asthma sufferers experience difficulty in breathing because the air cannot pass through the narrow bronchial passages. During an asthma attack, the bronchioles can become clogged with mucus and the person struggles to breathe for air.

There are many causes of asthma attack including stress, allergens and food intolerances. Allergies trigger the production of histamine, which constricts airways.

Many aromatherapy books warn against the use of essential oils for asthma since asthmatics are very sensitive against fragrances and you might accidentally make the situation worse. The safest time to use aromatherapy treatments are in between attacks.

Best oils to use:

The Beginners Guide to Making Your Own Essential Oils
2nd Edition

German chamomile - It contains chamazulene, which inhibits the production of histamine.

Frankincense, rose and marjoram - These oils can encourage deep breathing that allows the lungs to expand.

Chamomile, lavender, geranium, marjoram and rose

Lavender - You can use lavender steam to help open airways and to make the asthma attack less severe. You can also use an aromatherapy diffuser instead.

Pimple Treatment

Acne may not be considered as a health hazard, but it can affect your self-esteem and confidence. Acne occurs when the skin has been clogged with oil and dead skin cells. Bacteria feed on the oil that can ultimately lead to acne. People with an oily skin are more prone to acne.

Fortunately, many essential oils can help you deal with acne. Essential oils can balance hormones, improve completion and regulate the natural production of oil.

An essential oil compress is great to add to your acne regimen. You can make spot treatments, cream and even moisturizer with essential oils to help you control breakouts.

Best oils to use:

Tea tree - Tea tree is known for its antibacterial benefits. It can help kill pimple-causing bacteria.

The Beginners Guide to Making Your Own Essential Oils
2nd Edition

Neroli - It is great to use for mature, oily and sensitive skin. It can also help rejuvenate the skin and smooth out fine lines. It contains citral, which is a chemical that can regenerate cells and help prevent scaring due to acne.

Lavender - Lavender has potent antibacterial properties that can help reduce acne. It also has soothing properties that can reduce irritation and redness.

Rosewood - This oil is great to use on excessively oily skin. It can reduce sebum production and limit breakouts that are triggered by oily skin.

Bergamot - Bergamot oil blends well with other acne-fighting essential oils. It also has antibacterial and drying properties that make it a wonderful spot treatment.

Burn Treatment

The first thing that you need to do to cure minor burns is to submerge it in cold water mixed with essential oils. Remember that burned skin is very sensitive so it is better if you spray the treatment instead of rubbing it on.

Best oils to use:

Lavender - Lavender is very soothing to burned skin. It can also help reduce inflammation and decrease the pain.

Chamomile - It has skin-soothing effects that can heal damaged skin.

Comfrey - It has medicinal benefits that can reduce the pain caused by burns.

The Beginners Guide to Making Your Own Essential Oils
2nd Edition

Calendula - It is very effective in reducing burns because of its antioxidant properties.

Congestion Treatment

The most common trigger for sinus and lung congestion is flu or cold. Bacteria build up in the bronchial tubes can also help reduce irritation in the respiratory tract. If you want quick relief from congestion, then you can use peppermint, bergamot and eucalyptus and inhale the steam. The steam helps to open up the bronchial passages and lets the oil kill the bacterial infection.

Best oils to use:

Eucalyptus - Studies show that eucalyptus oil can help kill 70% of staphylococcus bacteria that can cause several problems.

Anise and peppermint - It helps relieve coughing.

Cypress oil - This essential oil can relieve runny nose.

Tea tree - Tea tree oil is effective in relieving congestion caused by bacteria. It has amazing antibacterial and antimicrobial properties that can help with congestion.

Earache Treatment

An infection usually causes earaches. While you cannot completely treat the condition by using essential oils alone, it can help improve the results drastically and can complement with other treatments.

The Beginners Guide to Making Your Own Essential Oils
2nd Edition

For a quick treatment, dilute lavender oil and tea tree oil with carrier oil and rub it outside the ear and along the lymph nodes on the side of the neck. Avoid putting it on the inside of the ear. Make sure that you use the treatment on both ears even if only one of them hurts.

Best oils to use:

Tea tree - Its healing and antibacterial properties can kill the main cause of infection.

Lavender - It helps reduce the inflammation.

Eye Strain Treatment

Long hours of exposure to computers can cause eyestrain. You cannot directly drop essential oil in your eyes, but you can apply treatment using a cold or warm compress. A warm compress is best for eyestrain while a cold compress can reduce redness and puffiness.

Best oils to use:

Lavender and chamomile - These oils can help reduce swelling in the eye area.

Insect Bites Treatment

Mosquito and other insect bites can be very uncomfortable when left untreated. A simple application of essential oils can help provide relief from itching. You can also add bentonite clay with essential oils. As the clay dried, it absorbs the toxins in the skin and prevents it from spreading further.

The Beginners Guide to Making Your Own Essential Oils
2nd Edition

Best oils to use:

Tea tree oil - It can disinfect the insect bite and prevent it from spreading further. Tea tree oil can also help relieve itchiness.

Lavender and chamomile - It helps swelling and inflammation.

Joint Pain Relief

Rubbing essential oil blends into the skin can help relieve muscle and joint pain. Remember to dilute your essential oil with alcohol or other carrier oil.

Best oils to use:

Cinnamon, clove and peppermint - These oils provide a heating benefit. This can stimulate the nerve endings and help relieve pain.

Rosemary, lavender and marjoram - These oils penetrate the skin and work on the muscles directly. It can also reduce inflammation and promotes muscle relaxation.

Chamomile, marjoram, birch and ginger - These oils are great to use for rheumatism and arthritis.

Indigestion Treatment

Digestive problems can be remedied using aromatherapy. Massaging essential oil blends in the stomach is great for

The Beginners Guide to Making Your Own Essential Oils 2nd Edition

children who do not like to swallow medicine. Also, do not undermine the effects of stress on the digestive system. Too much stress can impede the flow of digestive juices in the digestive organs. Too much tension in the stomach can lead to ulcer and colitis.

Essential oil can signal the brain that food is coming. This leads to the release of digestive juices in the stomach and small intestines. You can aid digestion by adding spices like caraway, anise, coriander and basil. You can also try drinking chamomile, lemon balm and thyme tea.

Best oils to use:

Peppermint, ginger, coriander, fennel and dill oil - These oils help relieve intestinal gas and stimulate appetite.

Rosemary - This oil helps in food absorption.

Peppermint - Peppermint can help treat bowel syndrome.

Lemongrass - This essential oil usually relieves nervous indigestion. It can also help sooth stomach cramps.

Menopause treatment

Not all women experience menopause problems, but those who do can find relief in using essential oils. It is usually used in combination with other natural treatments. Menopause syndromes include depression, hot flashes and confusion. You can apply the blend into your skin especially on fatty areas since this is where most of the hormones are stored.

Best oils to use:

Clary sage, fennel, angelica, sage, cypress, anise and basil - These essential oils have hormone-like compounds related to estrogen and can help relieve menopause syndromes.

Peppermint and lemon - Help reduce hot flashes.

Geranium and neroli - These oils balance hormones and can lessen the effects of menopause.

Nerve pain relief

The nerves are responsible for transmitting pain. Injured nerves may take a very long time to heal, but you can use essential oils to help with the healing process.

Best oils to use:

Chamomile, marjoram and lavender - These oils ease the pain of pinched nerves.

Helichrysum. This oil is specifically effective against nerve damage and can reduce painful shingles.

Poison Ivy Treatment

The extremely itchy rash caused by poison ivy can be very uncomfortable. It is best to choose essential oils that can reduce inflammation and reduce itching. You can also try soaking the affected area in an oatmeal bath.

The Beginners Guide to Making Your Own Essential Oils
2nd Edition

Best oils to use:

Peppermint - It contains menthol that relieves the burning and itching sensation.

Chamomile - It can reduce inflammation and stops the spread of the rashes.

Premenstrual syndrome treatment

Premenstrual syndrome or PMS is a condition that has many symptoms like headache, mood swings, irritability and water retention. It usually occurs 5-7 days before menstruation period. Aromatherapy can help with PMS in many ways. You can add the oils in your bath water or use it to massage your stomach area.

Clary sage - This essential oil can help with mood swings related to PMS.

Neroli, jasmine and rose - These have wonderful fragrance that can dispel irritability and moodiness.

Juniper berry, carrot seed, patchouli and grapefruit - These oils are great to use for excessive bloating and swollen breast.

Sore Throat Treatment

Bacterial infection or too much strain on the throat can lead to sore throat. The throat becomes inflamed, making it difficult to swallow. If your voice box becomes inflamed, then it can reduce your voice into a hoarse whisper.

The Beginners Guide to Making Your Own Essential Oils
2nd Edition

For several centuries, European singers are known for using essential oils and other herbal remedies to preserve their voices. You can also use diluted essential oil as a gargle.

Best oils to use:

Marjoram - It has antiseptic and anti-inflammatory benefits that can reduce bacteria in the throat.

Sage, thyme and hyssop - These oils can also reduce the effects of bacterial infection.

Lavender and eucalyptus - This can help you recover your voice.

Toothache Treatment

The main essential oil used for toothache is clove bud oil. Even dentists also recommend the use of clove bud oil. Make sure that the essential oil is taken from the bud and not the leaves because the lead contains eugenol, which is mildly toxic. You can also use clove bud oil to relieve teething pain in children. Remember that the clove bud can be hot so try it on your own mouth first before using it on small children.

Varicose Vein Treatment

Varicose veins occur when the circulating blood in the legs slows down. The muscles play an important role in circulating blood back to the heart. Varicose vein can be caused by standing for long periods of time and wearing tight pants that can restrict the blood flow to the pelvic area.

The Beginners Guide to Making Your Own Essential Oils
2nd Edition

The most common treatment for varicose veins is surgery, but you can also try essential oil blends to prevent the problem from worsening.

Best oils to use:

Cypress, palmarosa, myrtle, chamomile and frankincense - These oils can help ease inflammation and lessen the pain. These oils are also gentle on the skin so you can massage it in your legs.

Carrot seed oil - This oil specifically helps in skin conditions associated with enlarged veins.

Warts Treatment

Warts are raised areas on the skin. Human papilloma virus causes genital warts. You can detect genital warts by dabbing diluted vinegar into the area.

Best oils to try:

Tea tree and thuja - These oils are the best remedy for warts. Thuja is very strong so you need to dilute it properly.

Chapter 10

Create your Own Products Using Essential Oils

Learning how to make your own essential oil can help you save money in the long run. You can also use your essential oils to make beauty, body, homecare and pet products.

Hair and Scalp Products

Argan Oil Cooling Scalp Remedy

Healthy scalp can promote healthy hair. Peppermint and rosemary helps cool and invigorate the scalp.

4 drops rosemary oil

6 drops peppermint oil

1 oz argan oil

Add the peppermint and rosemary oil to the Argan oil one drop at a time. Pour in a dark bottle and roll it in your palms to mix. Apply to your scalp using your fingers. Rinse then style your hair as normal.

Sesame Oil Hair Protector

This hair serum can help prevent split ends and dry hair.

1 tbsp sesame oil

The Beginners Guide to Making Your Own Essential Oils 2nd Edition

5 drops clary sage

2 drops sandalwood

Simply combine all the oils together then apply on the scalp and into the hair shaft. Make sure that you coat the ends as well. Make sure that you use a few drops of the mixture at a time.

Shampoo for Dry Scalp

Relieve dry scalp and prevent dandruff with this essential oil shampoo

20 drops lavender oil

5 drops rosemary oil

5 drops palmarosa oil

10 drops carrot seed oil

5 drops sandalwood oil

2 oz unscented shampoo

Pour the shampoo in a bowl. Add the essential oils and stir before you transfer the mixture in a bottle.

Body Products

Chocolate Body Butter

Indulge your skin with this luxurious body butter. It is a great way to enjoy chocolate without the calories.

3 oz cocoa butter

The Beginners Guide to Making Your Own Essential Oils
2nd Edition

12 drops vanilla oil

3 drops tangerine oil

1 oz grape seed oil

3 drops ylang ylang oil

Melt the cocoa butter in a pot over low heat. Add the grape seed oil and stir. Remove the mixture from the heat. Add the essential oils then scoop the mixture into a jar. Allow to set overnight.

Tamanu Aftershave Lotion

Make this natural aftershave lotion to sooth your skin.

2 tbsp tamanu oil

24 drops patchouli oil

24 drops lavender oil

24 drops Roman chamomile oil

1 cup aloe vera oil

Mix all the ingredients in a bowl and stir gently. Scoop it in a dark glass container. Apply it to damp skin that has just been shaved.

Vanilla Body Moisturizer

This creamy body moisturizer captures the scents of vanilla.

1 cup cocoa butter

The Beginners Guide to Making Your Own Essential Oils
2nd Edition

1 ½ tsp vanilla oil

2 cups sweet almond oil

Place the cocoa butter in the freezer for 10 minutes. Transfer it in a small pot and melt it over low heat. Add the sweet almond oil. Heat it for several minutes until the mixture is liquefied. Remove from heat then add the vanilla oil. Let it cool then whip the mixture until it is soft and creamy.

Earthy Sweet Lotion Bar

This lotion comes in a solid bar. Your body heat will melt the lotion and make it easier to spread into the skin. The combination of the essential oils can make your skin silky smooth.

½ cup cocoa butter

2 tbsp macadamia oil

½ cup beeswax

2 tbsp castor oil

¼ cup coconut oil

½ tsp patchouli oil

½ tsp lime oil

½ tsp lavender oil

1 tsp vitamin E oil

The Beginners Guide to Making Your Own Essential Oils
2nd Edition

Cover your cupcake pan with liner. This makes it easier to clean up later on. Melt the cocoa butter and beeswax in the broiler method in medium heat. Add the macadamia, castor and coconut oil. Stir well to combine. Remove the mixture from the heat then add the essential oils. Whisk the mixture together and pour in the cupcake molds. This recipe will make 6 bars.

Lavender Vanilla Avocado Lotion Bar

This lotion bar is great for skin softening.

¼ cup beeswax, grated

½ cup coconut oil

½ cup cocoa butter

2 tbsp avocado oil

24 drops lavender oil

24 drops vanilla oil

Prepare a double broiler. Heat the cocoa butter and beeswax. Stir the mixture until it completely melts. Add in the coconut oil and avocado oil to the mixture. Stir the ingredients. Remove it from the heat. Add the essential oils then stir. Pour in your desired mold and freeze until it is set.

Foot Fetish

This refreshing foot spray is great to use after a long day.

5 drops rose absolute oil

The Beginners Guide to Making Your Own Essential Oils
2nd Edition

1 drop vanilla oil

15 drops sandalwood oil

1 drop sweet orange oil

6 oz water

Mix all of the ingredients in a spray bottle. Spray liberally on your feet. Cover with socks.

Cooling foot cream

This foot cream is beneficial after a therapeutic foot soak. It has delightful cooling effect that can relieve tired feet.

4 oz sweet almond oil

21 drops lavender oil

6 drops spearmint oil

½ oz beeswax

3 oz warm mint tea

9 drops peppermint oil

Place the almond oil and beeswax in a glass bowl and set it in a double broiler. Add in the warm tea to the oil and whisk the mixture to combine. Remove the mixture from heat. Submerge the bowl in a cool bath to make it congeal. Whisk the mixture vigorously. Add the essential oils and stir to combine.

Healing foot balm

The Beginners Guide to Making Your Own Essential Oils
2nd Edition

Pamper your feet using this essential oil foot balm blend.

¼ cup cocoa butter

2 tbsp macadamia oil

10 drops carrot seed oil

2 tbsp avocado oil

½ oz beeswax, grated

10 drops patchouli oil

Combine all of the ingredients except for the essential oil in a pot over medium heat.

Bath Products

Gentle exfoliating body scrub

Babao oil is great carrier oil for body scrubs. The invigorating oils can also perk you up in the morning.

4 tbsp sugar

9 drops tangerine oil

9 drops peppermint oil

1 oz baobab oil

Combine the sugar and carrier oil in a bowl. Stir until you have a pasty consistency. Add the essential oils. Apply the mixture on your skin to exfoliate the surface gently. Rinse off with water.

Mojito body Scrub

The Beginners Guide to Making Your Own Essential Oils 2nd Edition

This is a great body scrub to brighten your skin. The scent of the essential oils can also boost you mood.

3 tbsp sugar

1 tbsp jojoba oil

4 drops peppermint oil

1 tbsp grape seed oil

8 drop lime oil

Combine the oil and sugar in a bowl. Apply the mixture in your skin in a circular motion. Rinse it off with water.

Grey mood bath salt

Indulge in a relaxing bath using sea salt and herbs.

3 drops basil oil

3 drops sage oil

1 tbsp lavender flowers

3 drops rosemary oil

3 drops thyme oil

1 tbsp baking soda

1 cup sea salt

Combine all of the ingredients in a container. Stir to incorporate well. Use ½ cup of the mixture for each bath.

Mineral Bath

The Beginners Guide to Making Your Own Essential Oils 2nd Edition

This is a great recipe to emotionally uplift and soothe the skin.

2 tbsp baking soda

8 drops tangerine oil

8 drops chamomile oil

8 drops lavender oil

2 tbsp oatmeal, finely grounded

4 tbsp sea salt

Mix all of the ingredients together in a bowl. Add 2 tbsp. to your bath water.

Lavender Oatmeal Spa Bath

Lavender and oatmeal can sooth skin irritation and help reduce redness.

1 tbsp sea salt

1 tbsp ground oats

1 tbsp Epsom salt

27 drops lavender oil

Combine the ingredients. Add it to your bath water and soak for 10-20 minutes.

Lemon Bath Salt

The Beginners Guide to Making Your Own Essential Oils 2nd Edition

This simple and easy soap recipe is something that you can give away as gift. The lemon essential oil can invigorate the senses.

1 ½ cup goat's milk soap base

Zest of 3 lemons

6 drops lemon oil

Cut the soap base into cubes. Melt it in the microwave in two to three batches with one minute interval in between. Add the lemon essential oil once the soap fully melts. Stir the mixture well. Pour it into your soap mold and let it solidify.

Homemade energizing shower soap

The vigorous and aromatic shower soap has invigorating properties that can prepare you for the day ahead.

14 drops cypress oil

2 drops peppermint oil

8 drops lavender oil

4 oz unscented liquid soap

Add the essential oils to the liquid soap. Use it like any regular soap.

Spicy seduction body wash

Create a luxurious body wash with a romantic and floral essential oil blend.

The Beginners Guide to Making Your Own Essential Oils 2nd Edition

3 oz unscented liquid soap

1 drop clove essential oil

2 drops rose oil

3 drops vanilla oil

Combine oils in the liquid soap. Wash thoroughly with water.

Floral body wash

This easy shower gel also has moisturizing properties.

2/3 cup castile soap

1 tsp vitamin E oil

10 drop ylang ylang oil

2 tsp vegetable glycerin

2 tbsp honey

1 tsp jojoba oil

5 drops rose oil

Combine the ingredients in a bowl. Whisk the mixture vigorously until well combined. Scoop it into your container with a pump lid.

Beauty Products

Homemade facial moisturizer with SPF

The carrot seed extract provides somewhere between 35 to 40 SPF.

10 drops carrot seed oil

4 drops lavender oil

6 drops myrrh oil

4 drops frankincense oil

2 oz coconut oil

Combine the ingredients in a bowl and whip it until it has the consistency of frosting. Store it in a glass jar.

Radiant skin foaming face wash

Regularly cleansing your face with diluted essential oils can keep it radiant and smooth.

½ tsp sweet almond oil

10 drops ylang ylang oil

4 drops lemongrass oil

1/3 cup castile soap

6 drops patchouli oil

2/3 cup filtered water

Pour the soap and sweet almond oil in a foaming soap dispenser. Add the essential oils one drop at a time. Stir then add the water.

Facial serum with exotic blend

The Beginners Guide to Making Your Own Essential Oils
2nd Edition

Essential oils do not only smell great, they also provide wonderful skin benefits.

1 oz jojoba oil

1 drop rose oil

2 drops frankincense oil

2 drops sandalwood oil

Add all of the essential oils in a bottle with a dropper. Pour the jojoba oil gently. Gently roll the bottle in between your hands to combine. Use just one to two drops per application.

Healing scar cream

This healing cream is great to use for muscle and nerve damage. It can also help reduce skin inflammation

1 oz coconut oil

8 drops lemongrass oil

3 drops frankincense oil

10 drops geranium oil

6 drops lavender oil

3 drops rose oil

Place the coconut oil in a glass bowl and set over a pot of simmering water. Stir until it melts. Remove it from the heat and let it cool for 3 minutes. Add the essential oils. Stir the mixture and apply to the area twice a day.

The Beginners Guide to Making Your Own Essential Oils
2nd Edition

Skin calming face mask

This combination of clay and lavender essential oil can help calm redness and irritation.

14 drops lavender oil

1 oz bentonite clay powder

3 tbsp water

Combine all of the ingredients in a bowl. Stir thoroughly and apply on the face. Let it dry for 30 minutes then rinse off with water.

Geranium facial cream

Germanium oil is very nourishing to the skin. This cream is also a great makeup remover.

½ oz beeswax

1 oz rosehip oil

15 drops geranium oil

10 drop lavender oil

3 oz jojoba oil

3 oz distilled water

10 drops carrot seed oil

Combine the wax, jojoba oil and rosehip oil in a glass. Set it over in a double broiler method and stir until the wax fully melts.

The Beginners Guide to Making Your Own Essential Oils
2nd Edition

Add the water and whisk until you have a creamy consistency. Let the mixture cool then add the essential oils. Store it in a container.

Lavender & tea tree spot treatment

Jojoba oil is a nice to combine with tea tree and lavender oil since it does not clog your pores.

1 drop tea tree oil

2 drops lavender oil

1 tsp jojoba oil

Combine the mixture thoroughly and spread on the affected area.

Lemon skin brightener

Lemon oil has great clarifying properties and is great to include in homemade astringents.

3 drops lavender oil

3 drops lemon oil

3 tbsp water

Combine the ingredients and pour in a cotton pad. Spread it all over the face after cleansing.

Oily skin face mask

This recipe includes essential oils that can naturally dissolve excess oil. It also has a mild exfoliating effect on the skin.

3 tbsp white cornmeal

10 drop lavender oil

3 drops clary sage

3 tbsp raw almond meal

5 drops bergamot oil

3 tbsp water

Combine the almond meal and corn in a bowl. Add the essential oil. Add the water and stir until you have a creamy consistency. Apply into the skin in circular motion. Let it dry then rinse with water.

Revitalizing under eye serum

Making your own eye cream can be easy and inexpensive.

1 oz jojoba oil

2 drops carrot seed oil

10 drops rose oil

1 oz baoba oil

Blend the ingredients together and transfer in a dark colored bottle. Use your fingers to spread 1-3 drops under your eyes.

Macadamia & Rose lip balm

This lip balm has soothing and moisturizing properties that can make your lips smooth and plump.

The Beginners Guide to Making Your Own Essential Oils
2nd Edition

2 tbsp sweet almond oil

1 tbsp grated beeswax

13 drops rose oil

2 drops macadamia oil

¼ tsp vitamin E oil

1 tsp honey

Warm the beeswax, macadamia and jojoba oil in a pot over low heat. You can also prepare a double broiler if you wish. Continue to heat until the beeswax completely melts. Remove from the heat then add the essential oils. Place the bowl in a pan filled with cold water. Whisk the mixture until smooth. Add the honey and stir. Transfer the mixture into your lip balm container.

Cocoa & Chamomile Lip Balm

This nourishing lip balm is rich in healthy oil.

5 tbsp cocoa butter

1 tbsp argan oil

1 tbsp coconut oil

1 tsp honey

1 tsp unsweetened cocoa powder

3 tbsp beeswax

1 tbsp macadamia oil

The Beginners Guide to Making Your Own Essential Oils 2nd Edition

2 tsp vegetable glycerin

1 tsp vitamin E oil

25 drops roman chamomile oil

Place the beeswax and cocoa butter in a double broiler. Let the mixture melt thoroughly before you add the argan, macadamia and coconut oil. Mix the glycerin, vitamin E oil, honey and cocoa powder in another bowl. Stir well to combine. Remove it from the heat then add the glycerin. Whisk the mixture for one minute then place in a small container.

The Beginners Guide to Making Your Own Essential Oils 2nd Edition

Conclusion

Thank you again for purchasing this book!

I hope this book was able to help you learn how to make your own essential oil from scratch and know more about the uses and benefits of essential oils.

The next step is to start making your own essential oils and start living a healthier and stress-free life.

Finally, if you enjoyed this book, please take the time to share your thoughts and post a review on Amazon. We do our best to reach out to readers and provide the best value we can. Your positive review will help us achieve that. It'd be greatly appreciated!

Thank you and good luck!

The Beginners Guide to Making Your Own Essential Oils 2nd Edition

Check Out My Other Books

Below you'll find some of my other popular books that are popular on Amazon and Kindle as well. Simply click on the links below to check them out. Alternatively, you can visit my author page on Amazon to see other work done by me.

Coconut Oil for Easy Weight Loss

http://amzn.to/1i5f45p

Essential Oils & Aromatherapy

http://amzn.to/1ouuZTx

Superfoods that Kickstart Your Weight Loss

http://amzn.to/1eyHdku

The Best Secrets Of Natural Remedies

http://amzn.to/1gmHd7y

The Hypothyroidism Handbook

The Beginners Guide to Making Your Own Essential Oils 2nd Edition

http://amzn.to/1emWfyR

The Hyperthyroidism Handbook

http://amzn.to/1kqLQCp

Essential Oils & Weight Loss For Beginners

http://amzn.to/Q83bFp

Top Essential Oil Recipes

http://amzn.to/1lSrhSC

Soap Making For Beginners

http://amzn.to/1fkmYwr

Body Butters For Beginners

http://amzn.to/1fWjwJe

Homemade Body Scrubs & Masks For Beginners

http://amzn.to/1jjLRIO

The Beginners Guide to Making Your Own Essential Oils 2nd Edition

Carrier Oils For Beginners

http://amzn.to/1sbqUQP

Natural Homemade Cleaning Recipes For Beginners

http://amzn.to/1izDB2m

The Beginners Guide To Medicinal Plants

http://amzn.to/1vSujr6

The Beginners Guide To Making Your Own Essential Oils

http://amzn.to/1piUNSB

The Beginners Alkaline Miracle Diet

http://amzn.to/1sDVaVE

Thyroid Diet

http://amzn.to/1piW2RY

Essential Oils Box Set #1 (Weight Loss + Essential Oil Recipes

The Beginners Guide to Making Your Own Essential Oils 2nd Edition

http://amzn.to/1qlYWWP

Essential Oils Box Set #2 (Weight Loss + Essential Oil & Aromatherapy

http://amzn.to/1qlYWWP

Essential Oils Box Set #3 Coconut Oil + Apple Cider Vinegar

http://amzn.to/1oIFZJw

Essential Oils Box Set #4 Body Butters & Top Essential Oil Recipes

http://amzn.to/1jSxURJ

Essential Oils Box Set #5 Soap Making & Homemade Body Scrubs

http://amzn.to/RAvJYo

Essential Oils Box Set #6 Body Butters & Body Scrubs

http://amzn.to/RAvSel

The Beginners Guide to Making Your Own Essential Oils 2nd Edition

Essential Oils Box Set #7 Top Essential Oils & Best Kept Secrets Of Natural Remedies

http://amzn.to/1gvsRCq

Essential Oils Box Set #8 Homemade Cleaning Recipes & Essential Oil Recipes

http://amzn.to/1gxFAVb

Essential Oils Box Set #9 Essential Oil and Weight Loss & Carrier Oils

http://amzn.to/1jmcEPP

Essential Oils Box Set #10 Hyperthyroidism Manual & Hypothyroidism Manual

http://amzn.to/1nHgJU4

Essential Oils Box Set #11 Carrier Oils for Beginners & Coconut Oil for Easy Weight Loss

http://amzn.to/1nHfy6X

Essential Oils Box Set #12 Essential Oils Weight Loss & Essential Oils Aromatherapy & Natural Homemade

The Beginners Guide to Making Your Own Essential Oils 2nd Edition

Cleaning Supplies & Top Essential Oil Recipes & Carrier Oils

http://amzn.to/1nHfy6X

Essential Oils Box Set #13 Superfoods & Essential Weight Loss & Essential Aromatherapy & Body Butters & Soap Making

http://amzn.to/1nUds6v

Essential Oils Box Set #14 Weight Loss & Apple Cider Vinegar & Body Butters & Homemade Body Scrubs & Coconut Oil for Beginners

http://amzn.to/1i1qYOd

Essential Oils Box Set #15 The Beginners Guide To Making your Own Essential Oils & The Beginners Guide to Medicinal Plants

http://amzn.to/1m6wNC4

Essential Oils Box Set #16 Thyroid Diet & Hypothyroidism Handbook

http://amzn.to/1wmtIOI

The Beginners Guide to Making Your Own Essential Oils 2nd Edition

Essential Oils Box Set #17 Top Essential Oil Recipes & The Beginners Guide to Making Your Own Essential Oils

http://amzn.to/1BGYhBu

If the links do not work, for whatever reason, you can simply search for these titles on the Amazon website to find them.

Lightning Source UK Ltd.
Milton Keynes UK
UKOW03n1328270117
293041UK00002B/6/P